MATHA J. RUSSELL

The Whole Foods Diet

Delicious Recipes and Practical Tips for a Sustainable Whole Foods Lifestyle

Contents

Introduction

The desire to live a long, healthy life is as old as civilization itself. From Gilgamesh's mythological quest for the flower of immortality to today's pursuit of anti-aging medicines, the desire to avoid death and live a full life has been a consistent thread woven across human history.This yearning goes over cultures and generations. It can be found in the lullabies that parents sing to their children, the whispers of "many happy returns" on birthdays, and the quiet prayers for a loved one's recovery. It's a want to see the future unfold, to see children mature into adults and grandkids follow in their footsteps. It is a core human impulse, a primal desire to survive and enjoy life to its fullest.

Throughout history, the pursuit of longevity has taken several forms. Ancient civilizations sought mythological elixirs and miraculous herbs, while medieval alchemists worked in their laboratories to find the Philosopher's Stone, which was thought to bring immortality. With the growth of science and medicine, the emphasis switched to understanding the aging process and developing strategies to slow it down.Today, we are experiencing extraordinary medical advances. Vaccines have eradicated formerly feared diseases, and advances in treatment have significantly increased life expectancy. However, the quest for longevity is as strong as ever. We continue to push the boundaries of study, looking into subjects such as genetics and cellular rejuvenation in the hopes of discovering the secrets to living a longer and healthier life.

However, the aim of longevity should not be entirely based on the number of years lived. It is also crucial to examine the quality of life. A few extra years of life are worthless if they cannot be enjoyed. The actual goal should be to achieve healthy longevity, which is living a long life free of severe diseases while maintaining the physical and mental capacities to actively participate in the world around us. Adopting a healthy lifestyle that includes decent eating, frequent exercise, and appropriate sleep is the foundation for achieving long-term health. Furthermore, developing strong social relationships, participating in important activities, and maintaining a happy attitude can all contribute to a fulfilling and long life.

The desire for longevity is more than just a selfish want; it expresses our innate drive to positively contribute to the world, leave a lasting legacy, and make a difference in our corner of the universe. Living longer, healthier lives allows us to contribute more to our families, communities, and society as a whole. So, the next time you light a birthday candle, say a prayer for good health, or just think about the future, recall the everlasting human desire for long life. Let it be a reminder to not only aim for a long life, but also to make every day count by living a life full of purpose, passion, and joy.

Introducing the Whole Foods Diet: A Path to a Bright Future.

Imagine waking up every morning feeling energized, focused, and ready to face the day. Imagine a life full of vitality, good health, and a sense of well-being that emanates from within. According to innumerable individuals and a growing body of data, the whole foods diet has enormous promise.

The whole foods approach to eating is not a fad; rather, it is a shift in mindset towards supporting your body with its most natural fuel: unprocessed whole foods. Unlike fad diets, which emphasize fast cures and calorie control, the whole foods philosophy promotes a long-term commitment to eating for health and longevity. At its foundation, the whole foods diet favors whole, unprocessed ingredients over processed alternatives. Consider colorful and flavorful fruits and vegetables, whole grains such as brown rice and quinoa, which are high in fiber and nutrients, legumes high in protein and minerals, and nuts and seeds high in healthy fats and vitamins. Processed foods such as sugary drinks, processed carbs, and packaged snacks are reduced or removed completely.

But why did we pick this approach? The answer is found in the rising body of evidence indicating a significant correlation between whole meals and a healthy, vibrant lifestyle. According to research, prioritizing whole foods can:

- **Support healthy body weight:** Whole foods are low in calories and high in fiber, which contributes to feelings of fullness and promotes healthy weight management.
- **Reduce the risk of chronic diseases:** Whole foods contain antioxidants, vitamins, and minerals that can help reduce the risk of heart disease, type 2 diabetes, and some types of cancer.
- **Improve gut health:** Whole foods provide fiber and a variety of nutrients that help to maintain a healthy gut microbiome, which is necessary for digestion, immunological function, and overall health.
- **Increased energy levels:** Replacing processed foods with whole foods gives your body long-lasting vitality, allowing you to feel your best all day.

The whole foods approach is about more than just physical health; it may have a significant impact on your mental clarity and well-being. By providing your body with the best food possible, you may notice enhanced attention, mood, and vitality. Of course, following a whole-food diet does not imply perfection or deprivation. It is about making deliberate decisions, eating delicious and healthy meals, and living a sustainable lifestyle that nourishes both your body and mind.

Embarking on Your Journey: Understanding the Benefits and Setting Realistic Expectations.

The decision to adopt a whole-food diet is a step towards a healthier and more vibrant future. However, it is critical to approach this transition with both enthusiasm and realistic expectations.

Understanding The Benefits:

As you start, it's important to recognize the possible benefits that a whole foods diet can provide:

- **Improved physical health:** Whole foods are high in important nutrients, fiber, and beneficial chemicals, which can help with digestion, and gut health, and perhaps reduce the risk of chronic diseases such as heart disease, type 2 diabetes, and some types of cancer.
- **Enhanced energy levels:** Replacing processed foods with whole foods can deliver long-lasting energy, leaving you feeling less lethargic and more energized throughout the day.
- **Increased mental clarity:** Whole foods can help with cognitive function and overall well-being, including improving focus, memory, and mood.
- **Sustainable weight management:** Whole foods are often fewer in calories and more filling than processed foods, which can help with long-term weight management.

Setting realistic expectations:

While the potential benefits are enormous, it's important to set realistic expectations for your journey.

- **The transition may take time:** do not anticipate overnight miracles. Remember, a whole-food diet is a lifestyle change, not a fast fix. Be patient with yourself and acknowledge your minor triumphs along the way.
- **Challenges are inevitable:** Cravings, social situations, and navigating grocery shops stocked with processed foods are all potential obstacles. However, with planning and help, you can devise tactics to overcome them.
- **Focus on progress, not perfection:** Aiming for constant growth rather than absolute is critical. Slipups will occur along the road; this is completely normal. Don't allow setbacks to disrupt your progress; instead, resume with your next meal.
- **Celebrate non-scale successes:** Consider not only the number on the scale but also how you feel. Celebrate your improved energy levels, sleep quality, and overall sense of well-being.

Making Your Journey Successful:

Understanding the potential benefits and having reasonable expectations will help you succeed on your whole foods journey. Here are some more tips:

- **Begin small:** Start by making small, incremental modifications to your diet. Instead of going cold turkey, incorporate more whole meals into your daily routine while gradually lowering processed options.
- **Plan and Prepare:** To prevent making unhealthy choices while hungry, plan your meals and snacks ahead of time. Prepare meals at home whenever feasible to have more control over the ingredients.
- **Find your support system:**Surround yourself with others who share your health goals. Share your journey with friends and family, or join online communities dedicated to a whole foods lifestyle.
- **Enjoy the process:**Remember, eating healthy foods should be a pleasurable and enjoyable experience. Concentrate on learning new recipes, trying new flavors, and enjoying the satisfaction of nourishing your body with healthy nutrients.

I

Part 1: The Whole Foods Approach

1

Chapter One

Defining the Whole Foods Approach: What It Is and What It Isn't

Many people are turning to whole foods as a guiding concept in their quest for a better and more vibrant existence. But what precisely is it, and how does it differ from other eating trends?

At its foundation, the whole foods approach favors unprocessed, whole products over processed alternatives. This entails focusing on foods that are closest to their natural state, with minimal modification or processing.

Consider a bustling farmers' market loaded with fresh fruits and vegetables, stores stocked with healthful grains like brown rice and quinoa, and legumes like lentils and beans packed with protein and fiber. This is the essence of the whole foods philosophy: preferring natural, unrefined foodstuffs to packaged and processed alternatives.

Here are some major components of the whole foods approach.

- **Minimally Processed:** Whole foods are little processed, preserving their inherent nutritional and fiber content. Think about fresh fruits and veggies, whole grains, nuts, seeds, and legumes.

- **Nutrient-dense:** They are high in critical nutrients such as vitamins, minerals, antioxidants, and fiber, all of which are necessary for good health.
- **Unrefined:** Whole grains are consumed whole, with their bran, germ, and endosperm intact, as opposed to refined grains, which have had their nutrients removed during processing.
- **Closer to Nature:** Whole foods are closer to nature than processed foods, which are often loaded with added sugars, harmful fats, and artificial substances.

However, the whole foods approach does not involve imposing stringent restrictions or completely demonizing processed meals. It is primarily about making deliberate decisions and prioritizing natural, unrefined foods.

Here's what the whole foods approach is not.

- **A restrictive diet:** It's not about eliminating all processed foods or counting calories.
- **An overnight solution:** It is a long-term commitment to providing your body with nutritious ingredients.
- **Expensive or Exclusive:** It's about making thoughtful decisions and incorporating seasonal vegetables without requiring expensive or specialized components.

It's crucial to remember that the whole foods approach is a spectrum rather than a hard line. You can progressively adopt it and tailor it to your own needs and interests. Small modifications, such as replacing refined grains with whole grains or including more fresh produce in your meals, can have a huge influence on your health and well-being.

2

Chapter Two

Building Your Plate: Essential Whole Food Groups for Vibrant Health

The human body is a complicated and powerful system that requires several nutrients to function properly. While supplements can give focused support, nothing beats the power of whole foods to supply a varied spectrum of important nutrients and help you reach your best potential.

1.Whole Grains:

- **Nutritional Powerhouse:** Whole grains are high in complex carbohydrates, the body's main source of energy. They are also high in dietary fiber, which promotes gut health, aids digestion, and increases feelings of satiety. Furthermore, whole grains include vital vitamins and minerals such as B vitamins, magnesium, iron, and selenium.
- **Examples** include brown rice, quinoa, oats, barley, whole wheat bread, and whole wheat pasta.

2.Fruits:

- **Nutritional powerhouse:** Fruits are nature's treat, bursting with color and packed with important vitamins, minerals, and antioxidants. They are naturally low in calories and fat, making them ideal for maintaining a healthy weight. Fruits also help to keep your skin and eyes healthy.
- **Examples** include berries, apples, bananas, citrus fruits, melons, and tropical fruits.

3. Veggies:

- **Nutritional Powerhouse:** Vegetables are the hidden heroes of the plate, providing a diverse spectrum of vitamins, minerals, and phytonutrients, plant-based substances that promote health and wellness. Different colored veggies provide distinct benefits: green leafy vegetables are high in vitamins A, C, and K, whilst cruciferous vegetables such as broccoli and cauliflower are believed to combat cancer.
- **Examples** include leafy greens (spinach, kale), cruciferous vegetables (broccoli, cauliflower), root vegetables (carrots, potatoes), starchy vegetables (corn, peas), bell peppers, mushrooms.

4. legumes:

- **Nutritional Powerhouse:** Legumes, also known as "nature's multivitamin," are a nutrient-dense source of protein, fiber, vitamins, and minerals. They are an excellent plant-based source of protein, making them an important part of vegetarian and vegan diets. Legumes are also high in folate, iron, and potassium, which are essential for many body activities.
- **Examples** include beans (black beans, kidney beans, chickpeas), lentils, peas, and soybeans.

5. Nuts and seeds:

- **Nutritional Powerhouse:** These little nutritional powerhouses are packed with healthy fats, protein, fiber, vitamins, and minerals. Nuts and seeds are high in monounsaturated and polyunsaturated fats, which are good for your heart and help you feel full. They also include critical vitamins and minerals such as vitamin E, magnesium, and manganese.

- **Examples** include almonds, walnuts, cashews, peanuts, sunflower seeds, chia seeds, and flaxseeds.

6. Lean Protein Sources:

- **Nutritional Powerhouse:** Protein is an essential nutrient for tissue repair and growth, as well as muscle mass maintenance. While individual needs differ, including lean protein sources in your diet is critical. Lean protein sources provide essential amino acids, which are the building blocks of protein while containing less saturated fat or cholesterol.
- **Examples** include skinless chicken breast, fish (salmon, tuna), beans, lentils, tofu, eggs, and low-fat Greek yogurt.

Build a Balanced Plate:

Knowing the nutritional powerhouses within each food group is important, but learning how to construct a balanced plate is critical for optimal nutrition. Here are a few tips:

- **Half your plate:** Fill half of your plate with veggies that are not starchy, such as leafy greens, broccoli, or bell peppers.
- **One quarter of your plate:** One-quarter of your plate should be dedicated to whole grains such as brown rice, quinoa, or whole-wheat bread.
- **One-quarter of your plate:** Use lean protein sources such as grilled chicken breast, fish, or tofu.
- **Fruits:** Enjoy a serving of fruit with your dinner or as a healthy snack.
- **Healthy fats:** Eat healthy fats throughout the day, such as nuts, seeds, and olive oil, to maintain satiety and brain function.

Remember that this is a basic guideline, and your specific needs may differ depending on your age, activity level, and health goals. Consulting a qualified dietitian or nutritionist can assist you in developing a personalized plan based on your unique needs and interests.

Beyond the Plate: Additional Considerations.

While emphasis on full food groups is critical, the following aspects contribute to a healthy diet:

- **Hydration:** Drink enough water throughout the day to keep your body hydrated and support its numerous processes.
- **Moderation:** While entire meals are extremely nutritious, indulging in occasional pleasures is quite appropriate. Consume them in moderation while maintaining a healthy overall diet.
- **Cooking at home:** Cooking at home gives you control over the ingredients and allows you to produce meals from fresh, unadulterated whole foods.
- **Seasoning creatively:** Instead of using synthetic sauces and dressings, season your food using herbs, spices, and natural flavorings.
- **Read the food labels:** When purchasing packaged goods, pay particular attention to the contents and serving sizes, preferring those with identifiable whole food ingredients.
- **Support sustainable practices:** Support sustainable practices by shopping at local farmers' markets and selecting entire foods that are responsibly sourced.

3

Chapter Three

Understanding Macronutrients and Micronutrients: Fueling Your Body for Optimal Health

Our bodies work like complicated machines, requiring a variety of fuel sources to perform properly. Just like a car requires petrol to run and oil to keep its parts lubricated, our bodies need on numerous nutrients to conduct important activities, maintain energy levels, and promote overall well-being. These nutrients are essentially divided into two categories: macronutrients and micronutrients. Understanding their functions and incorporating them into your diet is critical for maintaining good health.

Macronutrients: The Powerhouse Provider

Macronutrients, or "large nutrients," are the foundation of our diet, providing the primary source of energy our bodies require to function. They are divided into three major groups:

1. **Carbohydrates:** Carbohydrates are often misunderstood or demonized, but they are necessary for supplying immediately available energy. They are converted into glucose, the major fuel for our brains and muscles.

Complex carbs, found in whole grains, fruits, and vegetables, provide long-term energy release, but simple carbohydrates, found in sugary drinks and processed foods, can cause energy dumps.

2. **Proteins:** Proteins, which serve as life's building blocks, are essential for tissue formation and repair, growth and development, and muscle mass maintenance. They are made up of amino acids, which are essential for many human activities. Protein sources include lean meats, poultry, fish, eggs, dairy products, and plant-based foods such as beans and lentils.

3. **Fats:** Despite being connected with weight gain, healthy fats are required for a variety of body processes. They offer energy, promote cell growth, aid in vitamin absorption, and help in hormone balance. Unsaturated fats, found in nuts, seeds, avocados, and olive oil, are helpful, whereas saturated and trans fats, found in red meat, processed meals, and fried foods, should be avoided for good health.

Micronutrients: the vital regulators.

While macronutrients provide the majority of our energy, micronutrients, or "small nutrients," play an important role in regulating a variety of body functions. They are required in smaller quantities than macronutrients but are similarly important for overall health. Micronutrients are further classified into two categories:

1. **Vitamins**: These vital chemical substances are required for a variety of body processes, including metabolism, immunological function, and cell growth. Different vitamins have distinct benefits, and deficiency can result in a variety of health concerns. Vitamin A promotes healthy vision, vitamin C improves immunological function, and B vitamins are required for energy metabolism.

2. **Minerals:** Minerals are essential for bone and tooth development, blood pressure regulation, and muscle and nerve function. Examples include calcium, which is necessary for bone health, magnesium, which supports relaxation and muscle function, and iron, which aids in oxygen delivery

throughout the body.

The synergy of macronutrients and micronutrients

Macronutrients and micronutrients work together to fuel our bodies for peak health. Here are some examples of synergy:

- **Carbohydrates and vitamins:** B vitamins are crucial for converting carbohydrates into usable energy.
- **Proteins and minerals:** Minerals like calcium and magnesium are essential for muscle function and protein synthesis.
- **Fats and vitamins:** Vitamin A needs healthy fats for proper absorption and utilization.

Build a Balanced Plate:

Understanding the relevance of macronutrients and micronutrients is essential for developing a balanced and healthy diet. Here are some suggestions for including them into your regular meals:

- **Include a variety of foods from each food group:** Fill your plate with a variety of fruits, vegetables, whole grains, lean protein sources, and healthy fats at each meal. This ensures you acquire a variety of critical nutrients.
- **Focus on whole foods:** Prioritise whole, unprocessed foods above processed alternatives. Whole foods contain a healthy balance of macronutrients and micronutrients, whereas processed meals frequently lack key nutrients and are rich in added sugars, harmful fats, and sodium.
- **Read the food labels:** Consider the macronutrient and micronutrient content of packaged foods when making purchase decisions. This information allows you to select options that are appropriate for your dietary needs.
- **Seek advice from a registered dietician or nutritionist:** If you have special dietary needs or concerns, seek personalized advice from a competent

practitioner on how to efficiently incorporate macronutrients and micronutrients into your diet.

Beyond the Plate: Additional Considerations.

In addition to integrating macronutrients and micronutrients through diet, several variables contribute to optimal health:

- **Hydration:** Drinking enough water throughout the day is vital for overall health and nutrient absorption.
- **Maintaining a healthy weight:** Maintaining a healthy weight lowers your risk of chronic diseases and allows your body to use nutrients more efficiently.
- **Physical activity:** Regular physical activity helps your body use nutrients more effectively, increases general well-being, and contributes to a healthy weight.
- **Quality sleep:** Adequate sleep is required for several biological activities, including nutrition absorption and metabolism.
- **Mindful eating:** By focusing on savouring flavors, recognizing hunger and fullness cues, and avoiding distractions while eating, you can make more educated food choices and maintain a healthy relationship with food.
- **Managing stress:** Chronic stress has an impact on your appetite, vitamin absorption, and general health. Find healthy stress-management techniques, such as exercise, meditation, or spending time outdoors.

4

Chapter Four

Shopping for Success: Selecting High-Quality, Whole Foods Options

Standing in the grocery aisle, overwhelmed by a sea of colorful packaging and unfamiliar labels, can be daunting, especially when navigating the world of whole foods. However, with a few key strategies, you can transform this challenge into an empowering experience. Here's your guide to choosing high-quality, whole food options in the grocery maze:

1. Prioritize the Perimeter: Most grocery stores strategically place processed and packaged foods in the central aisles, while the perimeters often house the fresher, whole food options. Make these areas your primary focus. Start with the produce section, selecting a vibrant array of fruits and vegetables in season. Look for locally grown options whenever possible, as they are often fresher and support local farmers.

2. Decipher Food Labels: While not foolproof, learning to read food labels can be a valuable skill. Look for the following:

- **Ingredient list:** This should be short and straightforward, with whole foods listed first. Avoid products with long lists of unrecognizable ingredients or added sugars.
- **Nutrient panel:** Pay attention to serving size, calories, and key nutrients like fiber, protein, and healthy fats. Choose options with higher fiber and lower saturated and trans fats.
- **Certifications:** Look for certifications like "USDA Organic" or "Non-GMO Project Verified" if these values align with your preferences.

3. **Embrace the "Less is More" Approach:** The simpler the ingredient list, the better. Opt for whole foods in their natural state, like whole fruits and vegetables, legumes, and whole grains. Avoid products with extensive processing or added ingredients like artificial flavors, colors, or preservatives.

4. **Befriend the Butcher and Bakery:** Many grocery stores have in-house butcher shops and bakeries. These sections often offer higher-quality meats and baked goods compared to pre-packaged options. You can ask questions about the source of the meat, cuts, and preparation methods, and inquire about the ingredients used in the bakery items.

5. **Explore the Frozen Section:** Frozen fruits and vegetables are flash-frozen at peak ripeness, preserving a significant amount of their nutrients. These can be a convenient and affordable option, especially when fresh produce is out of season or unavailable. Look for options with minimal added ingredients, like sugars or sauces.

6. **Embrace Imperfections:** Don't be afraid of "ugly" fruits and vegetables. These are often just as nutritious as their perfectly shaped counterparts and can be significantly cheaper. They are a great way to reduce food waste and save money while still enjoying the benefits of whole foods.

7. **Plan Your Shopping Trip:** Planning your meals and creating a grocery list beforehand helps you stay focused and avoid impulse purchases. This

ensures you prioritize your whole food options and avoid getting sidetracked by tempting processed snacks or sugary drinks.

8. Be Mindful of Marketing Claims: Companies often use clever marketing tactics to promote processed foods as "healthy." Don't fall prey to these claims. Focus on the actual ingredients and stick to your whole food principles.

9. Embrace Seasonality: Seasonal produce is generally fresher, tastier, and often more affordable. By incorporating seasonal fruits and vegetables into your diet, you can enjoy their peak flavor and nutritional benefits. Explore local farmers' markets whenever possible to support local farms and access a wider variety of seasonal produce.

10. Don't Be Afraid to Ask for Help: Grocery store staff, especially those in the produce and butcher sections, are often knowledgeable about the products they sell. Don't hesitate to ask questions about the origin, quality, or preparation of specific items.

II

Part Two: Putting It into Practice: A Roadmap to Success

5

Chapter Five

Planning Your Meals for Sustainable Change:Creating Weekly Menus and Grocery Lists

Going on a whole foods journey necessitates intentionality and planning, especially when it comes to navigating the world of grocery shopping and cooking tasty and healthy meals. Meal planning is one of the most effective success strategies.

Benefits of Meal Planning:

- **Saves Time and Money:** Planning your meals decreases the amount of time spent wondering "What's for dinner?" and eliminates last-minute grocery runs, which can often lead to impulse purchases.
- **Reduces Food Waste:** Planning your meals and purchasing certain ingredients will make it less likely that unwanted food spoils in your fridge.
- **Promotes Healthy Eating:** Planning ensures that you include a range of whole food categories in your diet, supporting balanced nutrition and assisting you in meeting your health goals.
- **Reduces burden:** Knowing your meals are prepared ahead of time minimizes the daily burden of determining what to cook, as well as the

temptation to choose unhealthy options.

Creating Your Weekly Menu:

1. **Gather Inspiration:** Look through cookbooks, culinary websites, and social media platforms for ideas. Consider integrating new recipes among old favorites.
2. **Consider Dietary Needs:** If you have any dietary restrictions or preferences, include them in your menu planning.
3. **Plan for Leftovers:** Leftovers can be repurposed into new meals for lunch or dinner, saving you time and decreasing food waste.
4. **Balance Variety and Simplicity:** Aim for a diversity of flavors and textures throughout the week, as well as some basic meals on hectic days.
5. **Consider Seasonality:** Choose seasonal vegetables wherever possible, as it is often fresher, tastier, and less expensive.

Developing Your Grocery List:

1. **Review Your Plan:** Go through your weekly plan and make a list of all the ingredients you'll need, being careful to measure everything accurately to avoid overbuying.
2. **Check your pantry and refrigerator:** Take inventory of your existing materials to prevent making unnecessary purchases and to make better use of what you have.
3. **Focus on Whole Foods:** Prioritise whole foods such as fruits, vegetables, whole grains, legumes, and lean proteins.
4. **Plan For Healthy Snacks:** Include nutritious snacks such as fruits, almonds, or yogurt to avoid eating bad foods during the week.
5. **Stick to the list:** Once your list is complete, resist the temptation to deviate while shopping.

Additional Tips for Success:

- **Cook in batches:** On the weekend, make larger servings of particular meals, allowing for easy and healthful leftovers all week.
- **Involve the family:** Get your family engaged in meal planning by encouraging them to offer ideas and help with the preparation.
- **Be flexible:** Don't be scared to update your meal or grocery list as needed due to unanticipated changes or item availability.

6

Chapter Six

Recipe Inspiration for Every Meal: Delicious and Nutritious Dishes for a Whole Foods Lifestyle

Embracing a whole foods lifestyle does not imply compromising flavor or variety in your meals. In reality, discovering the world of whole foods leads to a gastronomic experience filled with tasty and nutritious options for breakfast, lunch, dinner, and snacks.

Breakfast:

- **Power Smoothie Bowl:** For a creamy, protein-rich breakfast, combine frozen berries, spinach, Greek yogurt, a splash of almond milk, and a scoop of protein powder. Add granola, chopped almonds, and chia seeds for texture and flavor.
- **Scrambled Eggs with Smoked Salmon and Avocado Toast:** Prepare fluffy scrambled eggs with chopped fresh herbs. Toast whole-wheat bread and top with mashed avocado, smoked salmon pieces, a squeeze of lemon juice, and a sprinkling of red pepper flakes for a filling and savory breakfast.
- **Overnight Oats with Chia Seeds and Fruit:** Mix rolled oats, chia seeds, almond milk, and a touch of honey. Refrigerate overnight. Top with fresh

fruit, such as berries, sliced banana, or mango, for a cool and refreshing breakfast on the road.

Lunch:

- **Quinoa Salad with Grilled Chicken and Roasted Vegetables:** This flexible salad contains plenty of protein, fiber, and minerals. Cook quinoa, grill chicken breast, and roast your favorite veggies, such as broccoli, peppers, and onions. Combine with a simple vinaigrette dressing for a light and filling meal.
- **Chickpea Salad Sandwich on Whole Wheat Bread:** Mash-cooked chickpeas with celery, red onion, fresh herbs, and a delicious dressing of lemon juice, Dijon mustard, and Greek yogurt. Spread over whole-wheat bread and top with lettuce and tomato for a tasty and protein-packed vegetarian meal.
- **Lentil Soup and Whole Wheat Bread:** This thick and fragrant soup is ideal on a chilly day. Make a broth with lentils, vegetables like carrots and potatoes, and your favorite herbs and spices. Serve with a slice of whole wheat bread for a filling and balanced supper.

Dinner:

- **fish with Roasted Sweet Potatoes and Asparagus:** Season fish fillets with olive oil, lemon juice, and your favorite herbs. Roast sweet potato wedges and asparagus with the fish for a simple, tasty, and nutrient-dense supper.
- **Chicken Stir-Fry with Brown Rice:** Marinate chicken breast in soy sauce, ginger, and garlic. Stir-fry a range of colorful veggies, including broccoli, bell peppers, and carrots. Serve with cooked brown rice for a protein-rich and delicious dinner.
- **Lentil Shepherd's Pie:** This vegetarian take on a classic is full of flavor and nutritious ingredients. Sauté lentils alongside veggies such as onions, mushrooms, and peas. Top with mashed cauliflower or sweet potatoes for a substantial and cozy supper.

Snacks:

- **Trail Mix:** Create your own nutritious trail mix by combining nuts, seeds, dried fruit, and a hint of dark chocolate. This homemade version lets you choose the ingredients and avoids extra sugars and bad fats.
- **Hummus with Veggie Sticks:** Made with chickpeas, tahini, and olive oil, hummus is high in protein and healthy fats. For a filling and nutritious snack, combine it with colorful vegetable sticks such as carrots, cucumber, and bell peppers.
- **Apple Slices with Almond Butter:** This classic combo is an excellent example of a healthy, filling snack. The fiber in the apple keeps you full, while the almond butter contains protein and healthy fats.

Additional Ideas for Recipe Inspiration:

- **Explore cookbooks and online resources:** There are numerous cookbooks and websites devoted to whole food recipes. To keep your meals interesting, try different cuisines and flavors.
- **Seek inspiration from seasonal ingredients:** Choosing seasonal fruits and vegetables frequently means they are at their freshest and most flavorful. Use fresh food to create colorful and delicious dinners.
- **Get creative in the kitchen:** Don't be afraid to experiment and change recipes to fit your tastes and dietary requirements. Substitute ingredients, add your spin to existing recipes, and have fun discovering the world of whole-food cooking.
- **Focus on balance and variety:** Aim to include different food categories in your meals and snacks. This guarantees that you are obtaining the wide variety of nutrients your body requires to thrive.

7

Chapter Seven

Adapting the Whole Foods Diet to Your Needs: Addressing Dietary Restrictions and Preferences

The whole foods approach to eating focuses on eating unprocessed, entire foods in their natural state. While this idea has many health benefits, it is crucial to realize that one size does not fit all. Individuals' dietary demands and preferences vary depending on allergies, intolerances, cultural backgrounds, and ethical issues.

Understanding Your Start Point:

Before making any dietary changes, contact with a healthcare provider or certified nutritionist. They can evaluate your specific demands, existing health conditions, and potential weaknesses to provide a safe and personalized approach.

Addressing dietary restrictions:

Many people have food restrictions owing to allergies, intolerances, or medical issues. Adapting the whole foods strategy for these folks entails identifying suitable replacements while maintaining a balanced approach:

- **Gluten-Free:** If you have celiac disease or gluten sensitivity, avoid all gluten-containing foods, including wheat, barley, rye, and oats (unless certified gluten-free). Choose naturally gluten-free grains such as quinoa, brown rice, and buckwheat.
- **Dairy-Free:** Lactose sensitivity or ethical considerations may require a dairy-free diet. Replace dairy with plant-based alternatives such as almond milk, coconut milk, and soy yogurt. Ensure that these alternatives are supplemented with calcium and vitamin D, which are essential nutrients present in dairy products.
- **Nut Allergies:** If you have serious allergies to specific nuts, you must avoid them. Choose additional healthy fats such as avocado, olives, and seeds.

Catering To Preferences:

Beyond dietary constraints, people have personal choices influenced by their cultural background, religious views, or ethical considerations. The whole foods approach can be modified to fit various preferences:

- **Vegetarian:** Vegetarians can maintain a comprehensive and nutritious whole foods diet by consuming a range of plant-based protein sources such as beans, lentils, tofu, tempeh, and almonds.
- **Vegan:** Vegans who avoid all animal products can get enough protein from legumes, nuts, seeds, and certain whole grains like quinoa. Include a variety of veggies and fruits to meet your vitamin and mineral requirements.
- **Pescatarian:** People who eat fish can incorporate it into whole-food meals together with lentils, veggies, and whole grains. Choose sustainable and ethically sourced fish.

Maintaining balance and variety:

Regardless of your nutritional needs or preferences, keep in mind that balance and variety are fundamental principles of the whole foods approach. Ensure that your meals contain all key dietary groups:

- **Fruits and vegetables:** Aim for a rainbow of colors to benefit from the various vitamins, minerals, and antioxidants they contain.
- **Whole Grains:** Whole grains, such as brown rice, quinoa, and oats, provide more sustained energy and fiber than refined grains.
- **Lean Protein:** Choose protein sources from whole foods such as legumes, nuts, seeds, seafood, or lean meat (depending on your dietary preferences).
- **Healthy Fats:** To promote satiety and nutritional absorption, incorporate healthy fats like avocado, olive oil, nuts, and seeds.

Additional Tips for Successful Adaptation:

- **Read Food Labels Carefully:** This is critical for identifying potential allergens, added sugars, and hidden sources of undesirable components.
- **Embrace cooking at home:** Preparing your meals allows you to control the ingredients and ensure they meet your nutritional demands and tastes.
- **Explore New Whole Foods:** Don't be scared to try different whole foods to discover new flavors and culinary possibilities.
- **Seek guidance:** Consult a trained dietician or healthcare professional for personalized advice and assistance along your journey.

8

Chapter Eight

Overcoming Challenges and Staying Motivated: Practical Tips for Long-Term Adherence

S tarting a new lifestyle, especially one that requires dietary changes, might be thrilling at first. However, initial enthusiasm can fade over time, resulting in problems and potential setbacks. Staying motivated and overcoming these challenges are critical for long–term success.

Understanding the challenges:

Recognizing the most common obstacles people face is the first step towards overcoming them. Here are some common hurdles you may encounter:

- **Cravings:** Switching from familiar, processed foods to whole foods can cause cravings at first. These are only momentary reminders of your previous eating patterns, which may be dealt with with good coping techniques.
- **Social Pressure:** Navigating social environments where unhealthy food options are prominent can be challenging.The Chinese phrase (xuéhuì) – (xué - to learn, huì - to comprehend/master) - means "to learn and

understand" and can be used here. Learn and implement tactics for politely declining unhealthy options and suggesting healthier alternatives.

- **Lack of time:** When you're short on time, it might be difficult to prepare nutritious meals. Planning meals and grocery lists ahead of time, using quick and easy recipes, and integrating leftovers are all good techniques for dealing with this difficulty.
- **Motivation Loss:** It can be tough to stay motivated, especially when you reach a plateau or experience setbacks. Focusing on non-scale triumphs such as increased energy, better sleep, or strength will help keep you motivated.

Tips to Stay Motivated:

Now, let's get into actionable strategies to keep you engaged and committed to your journey:

- **Set SMART Goals:** Set SMART goals, which are specific, measurable, attainable, relevant, and time-bound, to provide a clear path for your trip.
- **Find an accountability partner:** Partnering with a friend or family member who has similar aims offers encouragement and support.
- **Celebrate Non-Scale Victories:** Don't just focus on the numbers on the scale. Celebrate increases in energy, happiness, sleep quality, and overall health.
- **Making Healthy Choices Easy:** To ease healthy eating, keep nutritious snacks on hand, chop veggies ahead of time, and use handy cooking options such as slow cookers.
- **Reward yourself:** Celebrate accomplishments and milestones with non-food rewards such as a new training wardrobe, a spa day, or a weekend getaway.
- **Focus on Progress, not Perfection:** Everyone faces setbacks. Accept them as learning opportunities and recommit to your goals.
- **Find Joy in Movement:** Experiment with various forms of physical

activity and discover new ways to enjoy movement, whether it's dancing, swimming, or hiking.

- **Seek assistance:** For personalized assistance and motivation, see a qualified nutritionist, therapist, or other healthcare professional.

Remember that consistency is crucial. Sticking to your new lifestyle for the majority of the time is significantly more successful than striving for perfection all the time. Accept the journey, be gentle to yourself, and appreciate your accomplishments, big or small. The key to long-term adherence comes in choosing a method that resonates with you and builds a lasting relationship with healthy living.

III

Part Three: The Whole Foods Diet for Specific Health Concerns

The Whole Foods Diet for Specific Health Concerns

9

Chapter Nine

Supporting Heart Health: Whole Foods Strategies for a Healthy Cardiovascular System

The human heart, a relentless engine that propels us through life, demands the greatest care and attention. Fortunately, dietary choices play an important part in maintaining its health and functionality. Adopting a whole foods approach, with a focus on unprocessed, nutrient-dense foods, is a potent method for maintaining cardiovascular health and lowering the risk of heart disease, the leading cause of death worldwide.

Understanding The Connection:

Diet has a substantial impact on heart health since it influences several parameters, including:

- **Blood Pressure:** Processed meals, which are generally heavy in sodium and saturated fat, can lead to high blood pressure, a key risk factor for cardiovascular disease. Whole foods are naturally low in sodium and high in potassium and magnesium, which assist regulate blood pressure.

- **Blood Cholesterol:** Consuming saturated and trans fats from processed and fried meals can raise LDL ("bad") cholesterol levels and contribute to plaque formation in arteries. Whole foods are often low in these dangerous fats and high in fiber, both of which help lower LDL cholesterol levels.
- **Inflammation:** Chronic inflammation promotes the development of heart disease. Whole foods high in antioxidants and anti-inflammatory chemicals, such as fruits, vegetables, and whole grains, can help fight inflammation.

Accepting Whole Foods for Heart Health:

Integrating these full food groups into your diet serves as the foundation of a heart-healthy plan.

- **Colourful Fruits and Veggies:** Aim to have a rainbow of fruits and veggies on your plate every day. They include high levels of antioxidants, vitamins, minerals, and dietary fiber, all of which are beneficial to heart health.
- **Whole Grains:** Opt for whole grains such as brown rice, quinoa, oats, and barley over refined grains like white bread and pasta. Whole grains contain complex carbs, fiber, and minerals that are vital for heart health.
- **Lean Protein Sources:** Choose lean protein sources such as beans, lentils, fish, chicken, and nuts. These meals contain needed amino acids for tissue growth and repair, as well as satiety management, which can help reduce unhealthy snacking.
- **Healthy Fats:** Consume healthy fats from avocados, olive oil, nuts, and seeds. These fats are required for a variety of human activities and can help enhance blood lipid levels.

Making heart-healthy swaps:

Simple modifications can have a major impact on your food habits.

- **Replace sugary beverages with water, unsweetened tea, or black coffee.**

- **Replace refined grains with whole grains. Choose brown rice over white rice, and whole wheat bread over white bread.**
- **Cook with olive oil rather than butter or other saturated fats.**
- **Choose lean protein sources such as grilled fish or baked chicken over fried or processed meats.**
- **Snack on fruits, nuts, or seeds rather than cookies, chips, or candy.**

Beyond the Plate: More Strategies:

While diet is important, a comprehensive approach to heart health is essential:

- **Regular Physical Activity:** Aim for at least 150 minutes of moderate-intensity exercise or 75 minutes of vigorous-intensity exercise per week.
- **Manage Stress:** Chronic stress might lead to heart problems. Use stress-reduction practices such as meditation, yoga, or spending time in nature.
- **Maintain a Healthy Weight:** Being overweight or obese raises your risk of heart disease. Maintaining a healthy weight via nutrition and exercise is critical.
- **Do not smoke:** Smoking is a significant risk factor for heart disease. Quitting smoking is the most crucial thing you can do to improve your heart health.
- **Regular Checkups:** Make regular appointments with your doctor to monitor your heart health, blood pressure, and cholesterol levels.

A Heart-Healthy Recipe Showcase:

To inspire your culinary adventure, here are some heart-healthy recipes:

- **Mediterranean Salmon with Roasted Vegetables:** This meal combines salmon, which is high in omega-3 fatty acids and good for heart health, with colorful roasted vegetables such as broccoli, peppers, and onions. Drizzle with olive oil and lemon juice for a tasty and nutritious dinner.
- **Lentil Soup with Whole-Wheat Bread:** This substantial and tasty soup

contains plenty of protein and fiber, all of which are good for your heart. Lentils are an excellent source of plant-based protein, while whole wheat bread has complex carbs and fiber.

- **Quinoa Salad with Chickpeas and Vegetables:** This protein-rich salad includes quinoa, chickpeas, cucumber, tomatoes, and bell peppers. Dress it with a mild lemon vinaigrette for a filling and heart-healthy lunch.
- **Fruit and Nut Trail Mix:** This compact snack contains a blend of healthy fats, protein, and fiber from nuts and seeds, as well as the sweetness and vitamins from dried fruits. It's the ideal heart-healthy snack for busy days.

Chapter Ten

Managing Weight Wisely: Utilizing Whole Foods for Sustainable Weight Loss and Maintenance

Weight management can be confusing, with contradictory approaches and alluring promises of rapid remedies. However, traversing this route necessitates a long-term and comprehensive approach that prioritizes not only weight loss but also general health and well-being.

Whole Foods Advantage:

Whole foods provide various benefits that make them effective partners in your weight management efforts:

- **Reduced Calorie Density:** Whole foods are often lower in calories than processed foods, which are often high in calories but low in nutritious content. This helps you to eat more food without exceeding your daily calorie limit, encouraging satiety and preventing overeating.
- **Fibre Powerhouse:** Whole foods such as fruits, vegetables, and whole grains are high in dietary fiber. Fibre is important for weight management

because it slows digestion, promotes fullness, and regulates blood sugar levels. This keeps you content for longer, reducing unwanted eating and cravings.

- **Nutrient Absorption Enhancement:** Whole foods provide critical elements such as vitamins, minerals, and antioxidants. These nutrients support your body's natural processes and promote a healthy metabolism, both of which are essential for weight management. Furthermore, a well-nourished body is less prone to seek junk food to compensate for nutritional shortages.

Creating a Weight Management Plate with Whole Foods:

To provide the groundwork for healthy weight loss, incorporate the following crucial whole food groups into your meals:

- **Colourful Fruits and Vegetables:** Try to have a range of colors on your plate at each meal. This rainbow not only adds visual appeal, but also provides a broad spectrum of vitamins, minerals, and antioxidants, all of which are beneficial to overall health and weight management.
- **Whole Grain Power:** Opt for whole grains such as brown rice, quinoa, oats, and barley over refined grains like white bread and pasta. Whole grains contain complex carbs, a consistent source of energy, as well as fiber, which keeps you full for extended periods.
- **Lean Protein Sources:** Include legumes, fish, poultry, and nuts in your diet. These foods contain needed amino acids for tissue development and repair, which promotes fullness and reduces cravings for harmful snacking.
- **Healthy Fats:** Consume healthy fats such as avocados, olive oil, nuts, and seeds. These fats are necessary for many body activities, including hormone balance and cell health, and they can also contribute to a sense of fullness.

Making Mealtime Modifications for Weight Management:

Simple dietary changes can have a huge impact on your weight management journey:

- **Portion Control is Important:** Begin by practicing mindful eating and controlling portion sizes. Use smaller plates to promote awareness and avoid overeating.
- **Embrace home cooking:** Preparing meals at home allows you to control the contents and portion amounts, ensuring that they are in line with your weight management goals. This enables you to make healthy choices while avoiding the hidden sugars and bad fats commonly present in processed foods.
- **Limit added sugars:** Added sugars in processed foods and sugary beverages are significant contributors to weight gain. Limit your intake of sugary beverages and instead drink water, unsweetened tea, or coffee. In addition, be aware of hidden sugars in packaged food and select options with lower sugar content.
- **Mindful Snacking:** While snacking can be beneficial, choose healthy foods such as fruits, vegetables, nuts, and seeds. Choose whole-food snacks that provide continuous energy and satiety over processed options such as chips, cookies, or candy, which can cause blood sugar spikes and cravings.

Beyond the Plate: A Holistic Approach to Sustainable Weight Management.

While eating is important, gaining and maintaining a healthy weight necessitates a comprehensive approach that tackles many elements of your life:

- **Regular activity:** Aim for 150 minutes of moderate-intensity activity or 75 minutes of vigorous-intensity exercise per week. Exercise helps to burn calories, build muscle, and enhance metabolism, all of which contribute considerably to weight management attempts.

- **Prioritise Quality Sleep:** Aim for 7-8 hours of good sleep per night. Inadequate sleep can affect hunger hormones, leading to weight gain. When you're well-rested, you're more likely to make good choices and resist cravings.
- **Manage Stress:** Chronic stress can impair weight loss by raising cortisol levels, which can lead to cravings for unhealthy foods. To maintain a balanced state of mind, use stress management strategies such as meditation, yoga, or spending time outside.
- **Stay Hydrated:** Drinking enough water throughout the day can help to reduce cravings, increase fullness, and promote overall health. Water also improves digestion and vitamin absorption, which are both essential for maintaining a healthy weight.

Whole Food Recipes for Successful Weight Management:

Here are some delicious and nutritious whole-food recipes to inspire your culinary adventure and help you achieve your weight management objectives:

Breakfast:

- **Overnight Oats:** In a jar, combine rolled oats, chia seeds, your favorite milk (dairy or vegan), and a sprinkling of cinnamon. Leave it in the fridge overnight for a creamy, fiber-rich breakfast. To add flavor and texture, top it with fresh berries or nuts.
- **Scrambled Eggs with Spinach and Tomatoes:** For a protein-rich and vegetable-packed breakfast, scrambled eggs with chopped onions, spinach, and diced tomatoes. Add a sprinkling of grated cheese for flavor and calcium.
- **Smoothie Bowl:** Combine frozen berries, banana, spinach, your favorite milk (dairy or plant-based), and a scoop of protein powder to make a colorful and tasty smoothie bowl. Add granola, chia seeds, and honey for an Instagram-worthy and tasty breakfast.

Lunch:

- **Quinoa Salad with Roasted Vegetables and Lemon Vinaigrette:** Combine cooked quinoa with roasted vegetables such as broccoli, carrots, and red bell peppers to make a colorful and tasty salad. For a refreshing touch, dress with a homemade lemon vinaigrette. Add grilled chicken or chickpeas for further protein.
- **Lentil Soup and Whole Wheat Bread:** This rich, warming soup is high in protein and fiber. Sauté chopped onions, carrots, and celery in olive oil, then add lentils, vegetable broth, and your favorite herbs and spices. Serve it with a slice of whole-wheat bread for a filling and balanced supper.
- **Tuna Salad Sandwich with Whole Wheat Wrap:** Choose a healthy and delicious alternative to regular bread. Combine canned tuna, diced celery, red onion, and a light mayonnaise or yogurt dressing. Spread it over a whole-wheat wrap and top with some leafy greens for added nutrients and a tasty crunch.

Dinner:

- **Sheet Pan Honey Garlic Salmon with Roasted Vegetables:** This simple but delectable dish is ideal for a hectic weekday. Toss broccoli florets, cherry tomatoes, and red onion cubes with olive oil and seasonings. Place them on a baking sheet beside salmon fillets seasoned with honey, garlic, and herbs. Roast them together in the oven for a nutritious and filling supper.
- **One-Pot Vegetarian Chilli:** This rich and savory chili is loaded with vegetables and beans, making it an excellent vegetarian alternative. Sauté onions, bell peppers, and carrots in olive oil, then add black beans, kidney beans, sliced tomatoes, vegetable broth, and your preferred chili spices. Simmer everything together until thick and delicious. For an extra protein boost, serve with a dollop of Greek yogurt and a sprinkling of shredded cheese.
- **Chicken Stir-Fry with Brown Rice:** This quick and versatile stir-fry is a nutritious and tasty dinner alternative. Marinate the chicken in a mixture

of soy sauce, ginger, and garlic. Stir-fried the chicken with a variety of chopped veggies, including broccoli, carrots, and bell peppers. Serve it with brown rice for a full and fulfilling supper.

Snacks:

- **Fruit and Nut Trail Mix:** This compact snack contains a blend of healthy fats, protein, and fiber from nuts and seeds, as well as the sweetness and vitamins from dried fruits. It's an ideal snack for busy days that is both heart-healthy and good for weight management.
- **Sliced Vegetables with Hummus:** Hummus is a tasty and nutritious dip made with chickpeas, tahini, olive oil, and lemon juice. For a tasty and healthy snack, serve with sliced vegetables such as carrots, cucumbers, and bell peppers.
- **Greek Yoghurt with Berries:** This protein-packed, fiber-rich snack is both tasty and filling. Combine Greek yogurt with your favorite fruit for a quick and nutritious snack.

Chapter Eleven

Boosting Brain Function and Cognitive Health: Whole Foods Choices for a Sharper Mind

Our brains, the constant command centers of our lives, demand the same level of attention and nourishment as any other critical organ. Fortunately, the foods we eat have an important role in maintaining brain function and improving cognitive health throughout our lives.

Understanding The Connection:

Diet and brain health are tightly linked. Foods contain vital nutrients that fuel a variety of brain functions:

- **Neurotransmitters:** Neurotransmitters are chemical messengers that allow brain cells to communicate with each other. Deficiencies in specific nutrients can impede neurotransmitter synthesis, altering memory, learning, and mood.
- **Brain Cell Health:** The brain requires certain nutrients to sustain and repair its cells, maintaining optimal function and cognitive health.
- **Blood Flow:** Proper blood flow to the brain is essential for providing

oxygen and nutrients. Some dietary components can help to enhance blood flow, which aids brain function.

Embracing Whole Foods for Brain Health:

Whole foods provide several benefits for cognitive health:

1. Rich in Essential Nutrients: Whole foods are naturally packed with vitamins, minerals, and antioxidants vital for brain health. They provide:

- **B vitamins:** Essential for neurotransmitter production and cognitive function.
- **Omega-3 fatty acids:** Play a crucial role in brain development, memory, and learning.
- **Antioxidants:** Fight free radicals that damage brain cells and contribute to cognitive decline.

2. Reduced Inflammation: Chronic inflammation is linked to cognitive decline. Whole foods generally have anti-inflammatory properties, helping to protect brain health.

3. Sustainable Energy: Whole foods provide sustained energy through complex carbohydrates, promoting focus and concentration throughout the day.

Making Food Choices for a Sharper Mind:

To nourish your brain, incorporate the following full food categories into your meals:

- **Colourful Fruits and Veggies:** Aim to have a rainbow of fruits and veggies on your plate every day. They are high in antioxidants and important elements that promote brain function.

- **Fatty Fish:** Incorporate fatty fish such as salmon, tuna, and sardines into your diet at least twice a week. These are good providers of omega-3 fatty acids, which are essential for brain function and memory.
- **Nuts and Seeds:** Make nuts and seeds part of your everyday routine. They provide healthy fats, vitamins, minerals, and antioxidants that are all essential to brain function.
- **Whole Grains:** Choose whole grains such as brown rice, quinoa, oats, and barley over refined grains like white bread and pasta. Whole grains provide prolonged energy and complex carbs, which aid with cognitive function.

Making Daily Swaps for Brain Health:

Simple changes to your food habits can make a major difference.

- **Replace sugary drinks with water or unsweetened tea.**
- **Replace refined grains with whole grains. Choose brown rice over white rice, and whole wheat bread over white bread.**
- **Cook with olive oil rather than butter or other saturated fats.**
- **Choose lean protein sources such as grilled chicken or baked salmon over fried or processed meats.**
- **Snack on fruits, nuts, or seeds rather than cookies, chips, or candy.**

Beyond the Plate: More Strategies for Better Brain Health:

While food is important, good brain health requires a comprehensive approach:

- **Regular Physical Activity:** Aim for at least 150 minutes of moderate-intensity exercise or 75 minutes of vigorous-intensity exercise per week. Exercise increases blood flow to the brain and stimulates the development of new brain cells.
- **Mental Stimulation:** Regularly challenge your brain with activities such as puzzles, learning a new skill, or indulging in creative pursuits.

- **Quality Sleep:** Aim for 7-8 hours of good sleep per night. Sleep deprivation impairs cognitive function and memory.
- **Manage Stress:** Chronic stress might cause cognitive deterioration. Use stress-reduction practices such as meditation, yoga, or spending time in nature.

Whole Food Recipe Showcase for Brain Health:

To inspire your culinary adventure, here are some recipes containing brain-boosting components.

- **fish with Roasted Vegetables:** This recipe contains omega-3 fatty acids from fish and antioxidants from colorful roasted vegetables such as broccoli, carrots, and bell peppers.
- **Lentil Soup with Whole-Wheat Bread:** This substantial and tasty soup contains protein and fiber, all of which are helpful to brain health. Lentils are high in plant-based protein, but whole wheat bread has complex carbs that provide long-term energy.
- **Berry Smoothie with Greek Yoghurt and Nuts:** This delicious smoothie mixes antioxidant-rich berries with protein and healthy fats from Greek yogurt and nuts, making it an excellent brain-boosting snack.

12

Chapter Twelve

Cultivating a Gut Microbiome for Optimal Health: The Role of Whole Foods in Digestion and Immunity

The gut microbiome is a varied ecology of billions of bacteria that live in our gut. This complex population of bacteria, fungi, and other microorganisms has a significant impact on our health, impacting digestion, immunity, mood, and metabolism. As research reveals the tremendous impact of the gut microbiota on our general health, maintaining a healthy and diverse gut ecosystem becomes increasingly important.

Understanding the gut microbiome's influence:

The gut microbiota performs a variety of important activities, including:

- **Digestion:** Gut bacteria break down complex carbs, fibers, and other nutrients that our systems struggle to digest on their own. This process enables us to take vital nutrients from our food and use them for energy and other biological functions.
- **Immune Function:** The gut microbiome works closely with the immune system to protect against dangerous pathogens and regulate inflam-

mation. A healthy gut microbiome can help avoid the overgrowth of dangerous bacteria and support a strong immune system.

- **Mood Regulation:** New research reveals a relationship between gut microbiome and brain health, with data pointing to possible effects on mood, anxiety, and depression.

The Power of Whole Foods for a Healthy Gut Microbiome

Whole foods provide various benefits for maintaining a healthy and diversified gut microbiome:

- **Prebiotic Powerhouse:** Many whole foods, such as fruits, vegetables, legumes, and whole grains, are high in prebiotics, which are non-digestible fibers that feed good gut bacteria. By feeding these "nourishing seeds," we encourage the growth and activity of beneficial bacteria, resulting in a more balanced gut ecosystem.
- **Diverse Nutrient Profile:** Whole foods include a wide range of vital elements, including vitamins, minerals, and antioxidants. These nutrients not only benefit gut bacteria directly, but they also improve overall gut health and function.
- **Promotes Gut Barrier Integrity:** The gut lining works as a barrier, keeping dangerous substances out while allowing necessary nutrients to be absorbed. Whole foods high in fiber and antioxidants can help preserve the integrity of the gut barrier, promoting overall gut health.

Creating A Gut-Friendly Diet with Whole Foods:

To cultivate a robust gut microbiome, include these whole food categories in your diet:

- **Colourful fruits and vegetables:** Aim for a variety of colors on your plate every day. This variant provides a greater spectrum of prebiotic fibers, which feed many types of good gut bacteria.

- **Whole Grains:** Choose whole grains such as brown rice, quinoa, oats, and barley over refined grains like white bread and pasta. Whole grains are high in prebiotics and fiber, which improve gut health and regularity.
- **Legumes:** Make sure to include beans, lentils, and chickpeas in your daily meals. These plant-based protein sources have high levels of prebiotics and dietary fiber, both of which are helpful to gut health.
- **Fermented Foods:** Add fermented foods like yogurt, kimchi, sauerkraut, and kombucha to your diet in moderation. These foods include live and active bacteria strains that can help maintain a diversified and healthy gut microbiome.

Making Everyday Choices For A Healthier Gut:

Simple dietary changes can significantly improve gut health:

- **Limit your intake of processed meals, sugary beverages, and harmful fats:** These can promote the expansion of dangerous bacteria and disrupt the gut microbiota.
- **Stay hydrated:** Drinking plenty of water throughout the day is essential for proper digestive function and gut health.
- **Manage stress:** Chronic stress can damage the gut microbiome. Use stress-reduction practices such as meditation, yoga, or spending time in nature.

Beyond the Plate: Additional Gut Health Strategies:

While diet is important, optimum gut health requires a holistic approach:

- **Regular Exercise:** Regular exercise is recommended to support gut health and general well-being. Exercise can boost good gut flora and lower inflammation.
- **Prioritise Quality Sleep:** Aim for 7-8 hours of good sleep per night. Adequate sleep is essential for a variety of physical functions, including

intestinal health.

- **Seek Advice:** If you are experiencing serious digestive troubles or suspect an imbalance in your gut microbiota, you should visit a competent healthcare expert for personalized counsel.

Whole Food Recipe Showcase for Gut Health:

To get you started, here are some gut-friendly recipes:

- **Lentil Soup with Veggies:** This hearty and tasty soup contains prebiotic fiber from lentils and veggies. It also contains plenty of protein and other necessary nutrients, which promote digestive health and overall well-being.
- **Yoghurt Parfait with Berries and Granola:** This breakfast choice contains probiotics from yogurt, prebiotic fibers from berries, and full grains in granola. This delicious and healthy mix boosts digestive health and delivers long-lasting energy throughout the morning.
- **Spicy Kimchi Fried Rice:** This tasty recipe combines fermented kimchi, high in live and active bacteria, with vegetables and brown rice, giving prebiotics and dietary fiber. To produce a balanced and gut-friendly meal, limit portion sizes and choose healthy protein sources such as tofu or chicken.

IV

Part Four: Living a Long and Vibrant Life: Beyond the Plate

Living a Long and Vibrant Life: Beyond the Plate

13

Chapter Thirteen

The Power of Movement: Integrating Physical Activity into Your Whole Foods Lifestyle

Modern living may often feel like a never-ending conflict between eating healthily and making time to exercise. However, in reality, these two components of well-being are inextricably linked. Adopting a whole-food lifestyle is incomplete without engaging in regular physical activity. It is a synergistic interaction in which each element enhances the benefits of the other.

Beyond the Plate: The Benefits of Movement for Whole Foods Eaters

Combining a whole foods diet with regular physical activity provides a powerful force for your overall health that goes beyond calorie burn. Here's how movement can help your whole foods journey:

1. Improved Nutrient Absorption: An active lifestyle promotes blood flow throughout your body, including your digestive tract. This enhanced circulation enables efficient absorption of critical nutrients from your whole-food diet. Your body makes the best use of the vitamins, minerals, and antioxidants you consume, maximising the potential advantages of your dietary choices.

2. Increased Energy: Whole foods deliver long-lasting energy from complex carbohydrates and healthy fats. Pairing this with regular exercise boosts your energy levels even more. Exercise strengthens your muscles and promotes cardiovascular health, allowing your body to use oxygen more efficiently and distribute it to your cells. This leads to feeling more energized throughout the day, helping you to take on your regular tasks with greater ease.

3. Improved Mood and Mental Well-Being: Physical activity is an effective way to improve mood and alleviate symptoms of anxiety and despair. Exercise causes the production of endorphins, chemicals recognized for their mood-boosting properties. Furthermore, the positive energy balance established via a combination of a good diet and exercise helps to improve mental health and overall well-being.

4. Stronger Muscles and Bones: Whole meals contain the necessary building blocks that your body requires to thrive. However, exercise is essential for muscle mass maintenance and growth, as well as bone strength. This powerful pair improves your physical abilities, lowers your chance of injury, and encourages a more active lifestyle as you age.

5. Weight Management Support: When combined with a well-balanced diet, regular physical exercise helps to manage weight and maintain a healthy weight. Exercise helps you burn calories, however, a whole-food diet guarantees that your body gets enough nutrients to support your activity level. This combination promotes a healthy calorie balance, allowing your body to function properly.

Finding the Movement That Moves You:

The secret to incorporating physical activity into your life isn't forcing yourself to do grueling routines you don't enjoy. It's important to find activities you enjoy and can easily include in your daily schedule. Here are some suggestions to help you start your movement journey:

- **Embrace the Outdoors:** Embrace the outdoors by going for walks, hiking, or cycling in nature. Immersion in the fresh air and natural environment enhances the enjoyment of your training program. Explore local parks, natural paths, or even your own home; the choices are limitless.
- **Discover the joy of dance:** Put on your favorite music and dance in your living room, or take a dancing class. Dancing is a fun and interesting method to get your body moving, and it is appropriate for all ability levels. Find what moves you, whether it's Zumba, salsa, or simply dancing to your favorite music.
- **Explore Team Sports:** Join a recreational sports team or find a group fitness class that suits your interests. Participating in activities with others develops a feeling of community, gives intrinsic drive, and can make exercise more social and pleasurable. Whether it's basketball, soccer, or a neighborhood fitness class, pick something that ignites your competitive or social spirit.
- **Make Everyday Activities Count:** Use the stairs instead of the lift, park further away from your destination, or integrate brief bursts of exercise throughout the day. Every amount of movement counts and adds to your overall activity levels. Squats while waiting for the kettle to boil, jumping jacks during commercial breaks, or parking farther away from the store entrance.

Making Movement a Habit:

Integrating physical activity into your whole foods lifestyle demands a long-term strategy. Here are some suggestions to help you turn movement into a valued habit:

- **Start Slowly and Gradually Increase:** Begin with manageable periods and effort levels that are appropriate for your *current* fitness level. As your fitness level improves, gradually increase the duration and intensity. Don't start severe workouts right soon because it might be demotivating and lead to injury.

- **Find an Activity Buddy:** Working out with a friend or family member can help you stay motivated and accountable, making exercise more pleasurable. Having someone to share the experience with can make it more enjoyable and help you stay focused.

- **Schedule your workouts:** Treat your workouts like important appointments, and mark them on your calendar to ensure they become a regular part of your agenda. Set aside a specific time in your day for physical activity, just like you would for any other important appointment. This allows you to prioritize movement rather than relying simply on current motivation.

- **Listen to Your Body:** Do not push yourself past your boundaries. Rest and rehabilitation are vital for avoiding injuries and staying motivated. Pay heed to your body's signals and schedule rest days as needed.

- **Celebrate your achievements:** Recognise and appreciate your accomplishments, no matter how minor. Milestones, such as finishing your first 30-minute workout or improving your running distance by a quarter-mile, need to be celebrated. Celebrating your accomplishments encourages great behaviors and keeps you encouraged throughout your path.

- **Embrace the Journey:** Remember that consistency is vital. Instead of random, hard workouts, aim for constant movement, even if it is only in small bursts throughout the day. The trick is to discover pleasurable activities that you can incorporate into your life daily, allowing you to gain the myriad advantages of movement while adhering to a whole-food lifestyle.

Movement and Whole Foods: A recipe for success

Integrating physical activity into your whole-foods lifestyle helps you to experience the full range of health benefits. Embracing activity not only maximises the benefits of your nutritional choices, but also improves your physical and emotional health. Remember that progress, not perfection, is the aim. Celebrate your accomplishments, rediscover joy in movement, and discover the transformational potential of combining a whole-foods diet with exercise.

Here are some tools to help you begin your journey:

- **The American Council on Exercise (ACE) website:** https://www.acefitnes s.org
- **The American Heart Association website:** https://www.heart.org
- **Centres for Disease Control and Prevention (CDC):** https://www.cdc.gov/ physicalactivity/index.html
- **The National Institute on Ageing (NIA) website:** https://www.nia.nih.gov

14

Chapter Fourteen

Cultivating a Healthy Mind: Techniques for Stress Management and Relaxation

In today's fast-paced world, stress has become an unwelcome constant for many. From tight job schedules and financial duties to juggling personal commitments and navigating a complex environment, our minds are continuously inundated with stimuli that can leave us feeling exhausted and depleted. However, building a healthy mind and properly managing stress is beneficial not only to our mental health but also to our physical health and general quality of life.

Understanding the effects of stress:

Stress is a normal response to difficult or stressful situations. It causes the release of hormones such as adrenaline and cortisol, preparing your body for the "fight-or-flight" response. While this response might be useful in some instances, persistent stress can have negative impacts on our physical and mental health, including:

· **Increased anxiety and depression**

- **Weakened immune system.**
- **High blood pressure and cardiovascular disease**
- **Headaches and muscle strain.**
- **Reduced sleep quality.**
- **Difficulty focusing and making decisions**

As a result, practicing good stress management skills is critical for preserving both mental and physical health.

The Power of Relaxation Techniques:

Fortunately, there are numerous ways available to assist us in managing stress and building a sense of peace and relaxation. Exploring these methods and determining what works best for you is critical to success. Here are some excellent ways you might implement in your life:

1. Mindful Meditation: Mindfulness meditation is the practice of focusing your attention on the present moment without judgment. This exercise teaches you to be aware of your thoughts and emotions without getting caught up in them. Regular meditation can aid with stress reduction, attention and concentration, and emotional stability.

How to Practice:

- Find a peaceful, comfortable area where you can sit or lie down without being bothered.
- Close your eyes or softly look down.
- Pay attention to your breathing, feeling the rise and fall of your chest or abdomen with each inhalation and expiration.
- If your mind wanders, softly return your attention to your breathing without judgment.
- Begin with brief sessions (5-10 minutes) and progressively increase the length as you gain comfort.

2. Deep Breathing Exercises: Simple deep breathing exercises can be a quick and effective approach to engage the relaxation response and counteract the fight-or-flight response that stress causes.

How to practice:

- Find a comfortable position, whether sitting or lying down.
- Put one hand on your tummy, the other on your chest.
- Inhale gently and deeply through your nose, and feel your tummy expand.
- Hold your breath for a few seconds.
- Exhale slowly with pursed lips, feeling your tummy contract.
- Repeat for a few minutes, concentrating on the sensation of your breathing.

3. Progressive muscle relaxation: Progressive muscle relaxation entails systematically contracting and relaxing various muscle groups in your body. This approach relieves physical stress and provides a deep sense of relaxation.

How to Practice:

- Begin with tensing and relaxing your toes. Clench your toes tightly for a few seconds before releasing and feeling the tension go away.
- Work your way up the body, tensing and relaxing various muscle groups including your calves, thighs, buttocks, stomach, chest, shoulders, arms, hands, neck, and face.
- As you relax each muscle area, concentrate on the feeling of tension leaving your body.

4. Visualisations: Visualization entails developing mental images of tranquil and calming places. This technique might help you shift your focus away from unpleasant thoughts and into a state of relaxation.

How to Practice:

- Find a peaceful, comfortable area where you can sit or lie down without being bothered.
- To relax, close your eyes and take several deep breaths.
- Imagine yourself in a serene and relaxing setting, such as a beach, a forest, or a mountainside.
- Engage your senses by imagining the sights, sounds, smells, and sensations of your preferred destination.
- Immerse yourself in the visualization, allowing yourself to feel calm and at ease.

5. Yoga & Tai Chi: Yoga and Tai Chi involve attentive movement, breathing exercises, and meditation. These techniques can help to reduce stress, increase flexibility and balance, and promote general well-being.

How to Practice:

- Consider taking a local yoga or Tai Chi class to learn proper technique from a certified instructor.
- There are also numerous online tools and instructional videos available to help you get started from home. For example, consider this meditation and yoga book with the ASIN: B0CTJ9YCQ6

Beyond Relaxation Techniques: Developing a Stress-Resilient Lifestyle:

While relaxation techniques are useful tools, developing a stress-resilient lifestyle entails more than simply managing stress in the time. Here are some more techniques to consider.

- **Regular Exercise:** Even 30 minutes of physical activity most days of the week releases endorphins, which are natural mood-lifters that can help with stress and anxiety. Choose activities that you enjoy, such as walking, swimming, dancing, and cycling.

- **Healthy Sleep Habits:** Aim for 7-8 hours of restful sleep per night. Establish a consistent sleep schedule, develop a calming nighttime routine, and keep your bedroom dark, quiet, and cool.
- **Healthy Diet:** A healthy diet includes nutrient-dense foods such as fruits, vegetables, whole grains, and lean protein. Processed foods, sweets, and caffeine should be avoided because they might worsen stress symptoms.
- **Maintain Healthy Relationships:** Care for your relationships with loved ones. Social support is vital for emotional well-being and can act as a stress buffer.
- **Connect with Nature:** Research has shown that spending time in nature can reduce stress, increase mood, and boost cognitive performance. Take regular walks through the park, go on treks, or simply relax outside and enjoy the fresh air and sunshine.
- **Limit Screen Time:** Excessive screen time can cause tension and anxiety. Set boundaries for yourself and restrict your screen time, especially before bedtime.
- **Learn to Say No:** Don't be scared to decline requests and obligations that consume your time and energy. Setting limits and prioritizing your well-being are essential for stress reduction.
- **Seek Professional Help:** If you are having difficulty managing stress on your own, do not hesitate to seek professional assistance. Therapists can teach you new coping strategies and offer support as you handle difficult situations.

Remember that maintaining a healthy mind and controlling stress are ongoing tasks. Experiment with different tactics, figure out what works best for you, and be patient with yourself. Prioritizing your well-being and adopting these practices into your daily life can help you develop a calmer, more resilient mind and negotiate life's challenges with greater ease and confidence.

15

Chapter Fifteen

Building a Support System: Finding Community and Encouragement in Your Journey

L ife's journey, whatever its objective, is rarely solitary. We all confront trials, celebrate achievements, and have periods of doubt along the way. Having a strong support system, or a network of people who offer encouragement, understanding, and assistance, can greatly improve our capacity to handle these varied situations.

Why Is a support system important?

Having a supporting network around you can provide several benefits, including:

- **Enhanced emotional well-being:** Sharing your joys and sorrows with other people can help you feel less alone and more connected.
- **Motivation and accountability:** Surrounding yourself with others who share your aims or values may keep you motivated and accountable, allowing you to stay on track and achieve your goals.
- **Practical aid:** Whether it's lending a listening ear, providing childcare, or

providing actual assistance at difficult times, a solid support system may alleviate your stress and allow you to focus on your journey.

- **Expanded perspective:** Meeting people with different origins and experiences can extend your perspective and provide vital insights, allowing you to negotiate complex circumstances with more understanding.
- **Reduced stress and anxiety:** Knowing you have someone to rely on can help you feel less stressed and anxious, allowing you to face obstacles with greater confidence and resilience.

Building a Supportive Network:

Building a strong support network does not happen overnight. It takes purposeful effort and dedication to form true connections with others. Here are some strategies to consider.

- **Identify your needs:** Consider what kind of help you require and what attributes you want in your support system. Do you need someone to listen and offer emotional support, someone to challenge you and push you outside of your comfort zone, or someone who can assist you with certain tasks?
- **Reconnect with old friends and family:** Often, significant support systems exist inside our existing social circles. Reach out to people you already know who share your beliefs and interests, whether to renew old friendships or deepen existing family relationships.
- **Join a club or group:** Participating in activities that correspond with your interests or aspirations can be an excellent way to meet like-minded people. Whether it's a reading club, a sports team, a volunteer organization, or a professional network, engaging with others who share your interests can lead to meaningful connections and a sense of belonging.
- **Be open to new experiences:** Getting out of your comfort zone and doing new things can lead to meeting new individuals. Take a class, attend a workshop, or volunteer in your community; these activities can help you broaden your network and meet people who could become key members

of your support system.

- **Be a good listener:** Creating a support system requires a mutual effort. It is not only about receiving assistance but also about providing it to others. Be a good listener, provide genuine support when necessary, and remember to return the compassion and care you receive.

Maintaining strong connections:

Creating a network is just the first step. Maintaining and cultivating these relationships demands consistent effort and attention. Here are a few tips:

- **Make time for your support system:** Schedule regular check-ins with your support team, even if it's only a quick phone call or video chat. Regular communication strengthens relationships and allows you to remain active in each other's lives.
- **Be genuine and honest:** Creating meaningful connections necessitates authenticity and honesty. Share your honest emotions, vulnerabilities, and joys with your support system so they may connect with the real you.
- **Develop individual relationships:** While group activities can be beneficial, it is critical to spend time developing interpersonal relationships within your support system. This allows you to develop a stronger relationship with each person and adjust your interactions and support to their specific needs and opinions.
- **Show appreciation:** Express your appreciation to your support team for their time, effort, and constant support. A simple "thank you" or tiny gesture can greatly enhance your ties.
- **Set boundaries:** Establishing and respecting personal boundaries is just as vital as making deep connections. Don't be afraid to say no when necessary, and prioritize your well-being.

Beyond Traditional Support System:

In today's society, support systems might go beyond traditional networks. Here are some more choices to consider:

- **Online communities:** Participating in online forums, social media groups, or virtual support groups related to your hobbies or aspirations can help you feel more connected while also providing helpful advice and encouragement.
- **Professional support:** Therapists, counselors, and life coaches can provide expert assistance and support while you work through personal issues and develop coping mechanisms.

16

Chapter Sixteen

Embracing a Holistic Approach: The Key to Sustainable Wellness

Our pursuit of well-being, a life full of vitality and fulfillment, is frequently a complicated road. We may focus on our physical health, going to the gym, and eating well, only to become bogged down by mental stress. We may pursue happiness, only to discover that it is transitory without a strong sense of purpose.

True, long-term well-being necessitates a holistic approach that recognizes and nurtures all aspects of ourselves: physical, mental, emotional, social, spiritual, and ecological. While each of these qualities is important in its own right, it is their interconnection that weaves the tapestry of a fulfilled life.

Understanding the dimensions of wellness:

1. Physical Health: This is the basis of our well-being. It includes healthy dietary habits, frequent physical activity, enough sleep, and preventative healthcare practices. Maintaining a healthy body provides us with energy, boosts our immune system, and improves our general quality of life.

2. Mental Health: Mental health refers to our emotional, psychological, and social well-being. It entails handling stress efficiently, creating happy emotions, and sustaining healthy relationships. Prioritizing our mental health allows us to face life's obstacles with more resilience and find inner serenity.

3. Emotional Health: The goal of this dimension is to effectively understand and manage our emotions. It entails recognizing our feelings, accepting their validity, and expressing them appropriately. By increasing our emotional intelligence, we can create healthier coping skills and strengthen relationships.

4. Social Health: Humans are fundamentally social beings, and our relationships with others are critical to our overall well-being. Our social well-being entails fostering ties with family, friends, and the larger community. Strong social relationships provide us with a sense of community, support, and affection.

5. Spiritual Health: This dimension refers to our connection to something more than ourselves, such as a religion, a sense of purpose, or a connection with nature. Cultivating a sense of spirituality can provide meaning and direction in life, promoting tranquility and well-being.

6. Environmental Health: Our surroundings have a huge impact on both our physical and emotional health. This component focuses on establishing a healthy and sustainable environment both within and outside the home. Toxin reduction, spending time in nature, and adopting sustainable behaviors all help to improve environmental health.

The synergy of a holistic approach

The beauty of a holistic approach is the interplay between these numerous dimensions. When we nourish them all, they help and reinforce one another, resulting in a cascade of positive effects. For example:

- Regular physical activity and a balanced diet not only benefit our physical health but also improve our mental health by elevating our mood and decreasing stress.
- Strong social relationships offer emotional support and can foster sentiments of belonging and purpose, which contribute to spiritual well-being.
- Practices that promote spiritual health, such as meditation or connection with nature, can help to alleviate stress and increase general well-being.

Integrating a holistic approach into your life:

Taking a holistic approach does not imply striving for perfection; rather, it entails making mindful decisions that promote your well-being in all aspects. Here are some ways to apply this technique in your daily life:

1.**Practice mindfulness:** Mindfulness entails paying attention to the current moment without judgment. This can be accomplished by meditation, yoga, or simply taking attentive walks in nature. You can make healthier choices that are better for your health by becoming more aware of your thoughts, emotions, and body sensations.

2. **Cultivate gratitude:** Expressing gratitude for the good things in your life regularly can considerably improve your overall happiness. Take time each day to think about what you are grateful for, whether it be excellent health, helpful relationships, or simply a gorgeous sunset.

3. **Prioritise sleep:** Adequate sleep is essential for both physical and mental well-being. Aim for 7-8 hours of sleep per night and stick to a consistent sleep pattern to ensure you wake up feeling refreshed and energized.

4. **Connect with nature:** Spending time in nature has various advantages, including reduced stress, improved mood, and increased creativity. Spend time outside whenever feasible, whether it's for a walk in the park, gardening, or simply relaxing beneath a tree.

5. Invest in relationships: Spend quality time with your loved ones, offer support, and show your appreciation. Strong social ties are critical to our emotional and mental well-being.

6. Develop a feeling of purpose: Identifying and following a life goal can provide meaning and direction. This purpose might range from personal ambitions and desires to contribute to a greater cause.

17

Conclusion

Key Takeaways:

Whole foods have potential: Consuming whole foods such as fruits, vegetables, whole grains, and legumes may help you live longer and healthier lives by minimizing cellular damage, supporting DNA methylation, and potentially lengthening telomeres.

Beyond the plate matters: A holistic approach to well-being is essential. Regular physical activity, stress management strategies, appropriate sleep, and strong social ties are all necessary for a healthy lifestyle.

Accept modest changes: Developing a sustained whole-foods lifestyle is critical. Begin small, investigate many possibilities, cook at home, prioritize authentic ingredients, and seek advice as needed.

Empower yourself: You can create a life full of meaning and well-being. Every conscious decision about food, movement, and self-care contributes to a brighter future.

Thrive, not merely survive: While longevity is important, the ultimate goal is to live vibrantly. Accept whole foods as a means of feeding your passions, building connections, and making a positive difference in the world.

Armed with these key takeaways and the knowledge you've gained throughout this book, remember: that you are the architect of your vibrant future. Every conscious choice you make, every step you take towards a healthier lifestyle, becomes a brushstroke painting the masterpiece of your well-being. Embrace the power of whole foods, not as a restriction, but as a liberation. Explore their delicious potential, and allow them to fuel your passions, nourish your spirit, and empower you to leave a positive mark on the world. Go forth, dear reader, embrace the journey, and thrive! May your life be a symphony of vibrant health, resounding with the echoes of your mindful choices and the joyful pursuit of a life well-lived.